Book Of The Best Skin Care For A Beautiful And Healthy Skin

Olatundun Solomon

olatundunsolomon@gmail.com

goodhealth1234567.blogspot.com

I have Honor Code Certificate from the University of Texas System edx. The course is 4.01x: Take Your Medicine-The Impact of Drug Development.

Am a Certified Alison Graduate with distinction in the course: Diploma in Nursing and Patient Care.

I have Honor Code Certificate from Harvard University through edx in the course PH201x: Health and Society.

Am a Certified Alison Graduate with distinction in the course: Diploma in Human Nutrition.

I also have Honor Code Certificate from edx Karolinska Institutet in the course KIBEHMEDx: Behavioral Medicine: A Key to Better Health.

It is good to have skin that is radiant and healthy. The skin can be free from pathogens (disease causing microorganisms). The skin can be beautiful and not have inflammation(dermatitis). The skin can be free from skin disease (dermatopathy).

This can be achieved by receiving the information of how this can be actualized. Hence, this book is very important for you to read. You will know the steps to be taken for you to have a beautiful and a healthy

skin.

The Skin

The human skin is made up of the epidermis(outer part) and the inner part(dermis). Blood vessels supply the skin in order for it to be nourished. The skin is used for the excretion of sweat. The skin take part in endocrine function by producing cholecalciferol, which is good for a healthy bone formation.

The skin is innervated, nerves carry sensory informations from the skin through the spinal cord to the brain.

The brain then interprets it and send the information back through the spinal cord. This makes the skin to be able to sense impulses of touch, normal condition, cold, heat and pain.

It is good to take good care of the skin. This is skin hygiene. Making sure the skin appearance is clean and free from germs is important. This makes the skin to look beautiful.

For the skin to be healthy, there are

requirements.

Ways Of Taking Care Of The Skin, To Make It Healthy And Beautiful.

Take your bath in the morning and in

the evening :

It is very important for you to take

your bath in the morning and in the

evening, this makes any disease

causing microorganism that may be present on the skin to be washed away from the skin. This makes the skin to be free from infection from disease causing microorganisms. This makes dermatitis (inflammation of the skin) to be prevented. Taking of bath in the morning and in the evening also prevent body odour. This is because the bacteria that will cause it is not present on the skin. This also prevent infection of the inner body parts, because the pathogens can not move from the skin into the inner parts of the body

to infect it with diseases.

Taking of bath brings the body

temperature to normal, this makes

the skin to be healthy because of the

normal temperature of the body.

Taking of bath makes the skin to be

soft and smooth, this prevent skin

wearing off.

The skin is very sensitive to the

environment.

For example, a job place that

produce glass, or asbestos. It is very

important to wear clothes that cover the body parts very well. This is because some thin particles from the machines that may be on the air will be protected from touching the skin parts that are covered by the clothes.

It is also good to wear helmet and spectacles for protection.

It is good not to allow acid to pour on the skin. Acid cause skin burn, this can damage the skin. It can make the skin to change color. It can

cause inflammation of the skin. It

can cause trauma to the skin. It can

even cause internal trauma to the

inner tissues of the body. Acid is

corrosive.

Sliced Green Cucumber:

Sliced green cucumber is good to be

rubbed on the face to treat pimples.

It prevent skin infection. It

moisturize the face.

It is good to be applied on the skin when there is dermatopathy(skin disease).

It treats skin infections.

It is used on skin discoloration

Eat Well Cooked Fish:

Fish has oil that has omega 3 fatty acid. This cause skin lubrication. This makes the skin to be radiant, beautiful and healthy. Fish is protein, it makes the skin to grow and develope normally. It makes worn

out tissues of the skin to be replaced

with healthy tissues.

Eat Lettuce As Salad:

Because of the presence of folate, it

helps in the production of

blood(hemogenesis) from the bone

marrow. This makes the skin to have

good blood supply. This prevent

unhealthy skin, by making the skin

to be well nourished. Lettuce also

has antioxidant that makes the skin

not to be damaged by free radicals.

Arrowroot treat acne.

Use Olive Oil To Rub The Skin:

This makes the skin to bc lubricated

and soft

This prevent wearing of the skin.

It makes scar to blend.

This makes the skin to be radiant.

This do not make the skin to break.

It do not make the skin to look dry. It moisturize the skin.

Olive oil is good to repair the skin.

It is used for skin cleansing.

It is used to heal traumatized skin.

Pomegranate is good to be used to make the skin to be repaired.

It treat fungi infection.

It is used as an antioxidant, it

protect the skin from free radicals.

It is antiseptic.

It is used on skin discoloration

Clary sage makes the skin to be

moisturized.

It treat acne.

Patchouli: It makes new skin cell growth occur. It is good to be used on skin that has experience inflammation.

Hazelnuts makes the skin to be moisturized.

Neem oil: It is used to treat bacteria infection.

It is used to treat fungi infection.

It is used to repel insects.

It is used to heal wound.

It is used to moisturize the skin.

It is used to treat pruritus(itching of

the skin).

It is used to treat skin inflammation.

It is antiseptic.

Manuka Oil:

Manuka oil is used to treat bacteria

infection of the skin.

It is used to treat fungi infection of the skin.

It is used to treat skin inflammation.

It is used to treat acne.

It is used for making the skin to be repaired.

It is used to treat itching of the skin.

It is antiseptic.

Myrrh is used to treat fungi infection.

It is antiseptic.

Neroli is used to treat fungi infection.

It is used to heal traumatized skin

Comfrey:

Comfrey treat inflammation of the
the skin.

It makes the cells of the skin to be in
normal shape.

It makes cell formation of the skin to
be normal.

Peppermint:

It can be used to treat acne.

It can be used as deodorant to make

a bacteria free environment occur.

Rub Sliced Aloe vera On The Skin:

This treat dermatitis(inflammation

of the skin) that is due to infection.

It also prevent skin infection.

This makes the skin to be healthy.

Aloe vera is good for skin repair after injury as occurred.

It makes the skin to be moisturized.

Aloe vera treat skin that has inflammation.

It treat acne.

It is antiseptic.

Elder flower treat skin inflammation.

It is used as an antioxidant, it

protect the skin from free radicals.

It is antiseptic.

It is used for skin cleansing.

Figs is used as an antioxidant, it

protect the skin from free radicals.

Lavender treat skin inflammation.

It treat fungi infection.

It is antiseptic.

It is used for skin cleansing.

Apricot kernel oil makes the skin to

be moisturized.

It treat pruritus(itching of the skin).

Apricot raw treat acne.

It is used as an antioxidant, it

protect the skin from free radicals.

It is antiseptic.

It is used for skin cleansing.

It is used to heal traumatized skin.

Blackberry makes the skin to be
moisturized.

Fennel makes the skin to be
moisturized.

Calophyllum is used for skin repair.

It is used to treat fungi infection.

Geranium is used for skin repair.

It is antiseptic.

Vitamin A is used for skin repair.

It is antiseptic.

It is used on skin discoloration

Drink Enough Water:

This makes the skin not to be

dehydrated.

It makes blood to flow normally in

the body.

It makes the skin not to break.

It makes the skin to be soft and

healthy.

It makes the temperature of the skin

to be normal.

Eucalyptus is good to treat bacteria infection. It is good to treat acne. It good to be used as antiseptic.

It treat acne.

It is used as insect repellant

EMU oil is good to be used to treat inflammation of the skin. It is also good to be used to treat bacteria infection of the skin. It moisturize the skin. It is good to be used on scar and stretch marks.

Gotu kola is used to treat blackheads.

It treat acne.

Egg white is good to be used to treat blackheads.

It is used for skin cleansing.

Banana It is used for skin cleansing.

Cedarwood It is used for skin

cleansing.

Evening primrose is good to be used

to treat blackheads. It is also good to

make the skin to be repaired. It

makes the skin to be moisturized.

It treat acne.

Safflower oil makes the skin to be

moisturized.

It is used as an antioxidant, it

protect the skin from free radicals.

Apple Cider is good to treat

blackheads.

It also treat pruritus(itching of the

skin).

It treat acne.

It is antiseptic.

Apple moisturize the skin.

It is used as an antioxidant, it protect the skin from free radicals. It is used for skin cleansing.

Vinegar can be used to treat blackheads.

It is also used to treat pruritus(itching).

It treat acne.

It is used as an antioxidant, it protect the skin from free radicals.

It is antiseptic.

It is used for skin cleansing.

Arrowroot is used to treat

blackheads.

Kanaja oil makes the skin to be

moisturized.

Baking soda treat pruritus(skin

itching). After treatment wash it

away with clean water.

Eat Slices Of Carrots And Tomatoes

as salad:

This as phytonutrients that makes

the skin to have positive health.

It has antioxidant that helps the skin

not to be damaged by free radicals.

There is lot of fluid in it, this makes

the skin to be hydrated, this makes

the skin to be fresh.

This prevent wrinkles on the face.

Have Good Sleep:

Sleep is very important to make the skin to be healthy.

This makes the skin to be refreshed.

This makes the circadian rhythm of the body to be normal.

This makes the heart, liver, brain and other parts of the body to function well in order for the skin to be healthy.

Exercise:

Exercise is very good for the skin to be healthy.

The sweating out makes the pores of the skin to be well opened, this refreshes the skin with environmental air.

It is good to bath after exercise, this prevent body odour.

Make Sure The Phone Is Clean:

This prevent infection by microorganisms from the phone surface.

This makes the skin to be free from diseases.

Eating Coconut:

Because of the oil in the coconut it makes the skin to be radiant.

It makes the skin to be moisturized.

It makes the skin not to break.

It has unsaturated fatty acid this

makes the body to have healthy skin.

is used as antioxidant to prevent

damage of the skin by free radicals.

Gooseberry is used as antioxidant to

prevent damage of the skin by free

radicals.

Licorice is used as antioxidant to

prevent damage of the skin by free

radicals.

Juniper makes the skin to be moisturized.

It is antiseptic.

Argan Oil:

Protect the skin from damaging due to the ray from the sun light.

It moisturize the skin, thereby preventing dehydration.

It treat psoriasis.

It treat acne.

It makes wound to heal.

It is good to treat pruritus(itching).

It is used as an antioxidant, it

protect the skin from free radicals.

Aubergine is used as an antioxidant,

it protect the skin from free radicals.

Shea Butter:

Shea butter is good to be rubbed on the skin.

It prevent skin breakage.

It moisturize the skin.

It makes the skin to be radiant.

It makes the skin to be soft and healthy.

It is good for skin repair after injury.

It makes the skin to be hydrated.

Rosehip Oil: It is good for healing injury.

It makes production of new skin tissue to occur.

It is good for making collagen production to occur thereby making repair and healing of wound to happen.

Rosehip oil makes the skin to be moisturized.

It treat acne.

It treat fungi infection.

It is used as an antioxidant, it

protect the skin from free radicals.

It is antiseptic.

It is used on skin discoloration.

Almond meal and almond oil makes

the skin to be moisturized.

Is used to treat acne.

Is used to treat fungi infection.

It is used as an antioxidant, it protect

the skin from free radicals.

It is antiseptic.

It is used for skin cleansing.

Sunflower Oil:

It has oleic acid.

It has linoleic acid.

It moisturize the skin.

It prevent skin breakage.

It is used as an antioxidant, it

protect the skin from free radicals.

Lanolin makes the skin to be

moisturized.

Wheatgerm Oil:

It treat inflammation of the skin.

It has vitamin E.

It treat eczema.

It treat psoriasis.

It is good to be use for the healing of

wound.

Meadow Foam Oil:

It moisturize the skin.

It is good to be used for treating

inflammation of the skin.

It makes the skin to be soft.

It prevent the skin from breaking.

Macadamia Nut Oil:

It has oleic acid.

It makes new cells of skin tissue to occur, thereby repairing injured skin.

It moisturize the skin, thereby preventing skin breakage.

It treat acne.

It makes the skin to be soft.

It makes the skin to be smooth.

It can be used to treat blackheads.

Carrot seed makes the skin to be moisturized.

It is used as an antioxidant, it

protect the skin from free radicals.

It is antiseptic.

It is used to heal traumatized skin.

Frankincense

Frankincense can be used on wound

in order to experience healing.

It can also be used to treat acne.

It is also good to be used for skin growth.

It is good to be used to moisturize the skin.

Hazelnut Oil:

It has vitamin A.

It has vitamin E.

It has vitamin B.

It makes the skin to be soft.

It does not make the skin to be dehydrated.

It is good for treating acne.

Basil is used to treat acne.

It is used for skin cleansing.

Guava is used to treat acne.

It is used as an antioxidant, it protect the skin from free radicals.

It is used for skin cleansing.

Karanja oil

Karanja oil is good to be used for bacteria infection.

It is good to be used to treat inflammation of the skin.

It is used to treat fungi infection of the skin.

It is used to repel insects.

It is used to treat pruritus(itching). It is good to be used to heal wound.

It is antiseptic.

Oatmeal is used to treat pruritus(itching of the skin).

It is antiseptic.

It is also used to treat psoriasis.

Bergamot: It makes new healthy skin to grow.

It makes wound to have healing.

It makes the skin to grow normally in a healthy way.

It treat acne.

It is antiseptic.

It is used for skin cleansing.

Grapefruit: It is good to be used as antiseptic.

It is good to be used to treat bacteria infection.

It is an astringent.

It is deodorant.

It is an antiseptic.

It is used for skin cleansing.

Lemongrass: It is antibacterial.

Camellia Oil: It has omega-9 fatty

acid.

It moisturize the skin.

It does not make pores of the skin to

block.

Do Not Stay Under The Sun As An

Hobby.

Staying under the sun as an hobby

can cause skin cancer from the ultra

violet radiation.

It can cause sun burn.

It can change the color of the skin.

It can cause dehydration of the skin.

It can make the skin to break.

It can cause wear and tear of the

skin.

Use Soy Oil To Cook And Drink Soy
Milk:

The soy milk is protein. This makes a good skin growth and development to occur.

The soy oil makes the skin to be radiant.

The soy milk as antioxidant, this makes the skin not to be destroyed by free radicals.

The soy milk moisturize the skin.

The soy milk hydrate the skin and prevent dehydration of the skin, this prevent the skin from breaking.

Add Thyme And Curry To Food When Cooking:

Thyme is disinfectant and curry is antibiotics. Thyme treat acne. It also treat bacteria infection. It treat rashes. It treat itching of the skin.

This makes the skin to be free from infection.

It makes any pathogen(disease causing microorganism) not to be present in the skin.

This makes skin hygiene to occur.

Honey:

Honey is antibacterial.

It can be used on fungi infection.

It can be used on skin inflammation.

It can be used on wound to heal it.

It can be used to make the skin to be
repaired.

It is used as an antioxidant, it
protect the skin from free radicals.

It is used for skin cleansing.

Acaiberry is used as antioxidant to
prevent damage of the skin by free
radicals.

Kiwifruit is used as an antioxidant, it
protect the skin from free radicals.

Melons is used as an antioxidant, it

protect the skin from free radicals.

Calendula is used to make the skin

to be repaired.

It treat skin inflammation.

It treat acne.

It treat fungi infection.

It is used to heal traumatized skin

Eat Avocado:

Avocado as enough vitamin K, this prevent blood loss, this makes the body to have enough blood to nourish the skin.

Avocado as enough oil to lubricate the skin. This makes the skin to be radiant. Avocado is good to be used for skin repair.

Avocado moisturize the skin, this prevent skin breakage.

It is used as an antioxidant, it protect the skin from free radicals.

Jojoba Oil

Jojoba oil is good to be used on the skin.

It prevent skin breakage.

It makes the skin to be radiant.

It prevent wear and tear of the skin.

Jojoba liquid wax makes the skin to be moisturized.

It treat inflammation of the skin.

It treat eczema.

It treat psoriasis.

It is used for skin cleansing.

This makes the skin to be healthy

and beautiful.

Don't Burse Pimples:

When pimples is burst by using the

fingers, it can cause spots on the

face.

Rub sliced cucumber and sliced lemon on the face, this will resolve the pimples.

It treat acne.

It is antiseptic.

Eat Peanut:

When you eat peanut it makes the skin the grow and develope well.

It makes the skin to be lubricated well.

It makes the skin to be radiant because of the oil in it.

It prevent skin breakage.

It prevent wear and tear of the skin.

Don't Put Too Much Sugar In The Food That Is To Be Eaten:

When too much sugar is in food, it can cause diabetes mellitus. This can cause traumatized (injured) skin to not heal quickly. This can result to other infections, because pathogens can use the breakage of the skin to

further increase the infection of the

skin.

Green Beans:

Green beans makes the skin to grow

normally and develope healthily.

It repairs worn out tissues of the skin.

The folate in it makes blood to be

produced from the bone marrow.

This makes the skin to be well

nourished and it makes the skin to

be healthy.

Acne Removal:

Acne can be removed by slicing

lemon and lime.

Rub on the part that is affected by

acne. This helps to remove it.

Blackheads Removal:

Slice lemon and lime.

Remove the seeds.

Squeeze the juice into the mouth and drink it.

This helps liver in emulsification of fat.

This makes blackheads to be resolved.

Drink green tea this also helps in the removal of blackheads.

Using lemon juice on the parts that has blackheads makes the blackheads to be resolved.

Cancer Of The Skin:

This can be resolved by drinking green tea. It has anticancer effect in it.

Cancer of the skin can be prevented by not staying under sun, by not sitting under the sun. This prevent ultraviolet radiation from affecting the skin. It is good to be protected from radioactive radiation.

Green tea is also used as antioxidant to prevent damage of the skin by free radicals.

It is used to treat acne.

It is used to treat rosacea.

Feverfew is used to treat acne.

It is also used to treat rosacea.

Pawpaw:

Eat pawpaw , it prevent skin from dehydration.

Eat pawpaw, it makes the skin to be soft and smooth.

Pawpaw has beta carotene, that helps in the formation of vitamin A in the body. This is good for a healthy skin formation.

Castor Oil:

It is good to use castor oil on the area of the skin that is infected by

pathogens (disease causing
microorganisms) e.g. eczema. It get
rid of it.

After using the castor oil wash your
hands with soap and water. It is also
good to bath after some minutes of
applying the castor oil on the
affected part.

Please note. Do not drink the castor
oil, because it is poisonous.

Cocoa Butter:

It is good to use cocoa butter on the skin.

It moisturize the skin.

It makes the skin to be radiant.

It makes the skin to be healthy.

It makes the skin to be beautiful.

It makes the skin to be smooth.

It makes the skin to be soft.

It protect the skin.

Arbutin is used as antioxidant to prevent damage of the skin by free radicals.

Burn On The Skin:

When there is burn on the skin use the liquid of egg and rub it on the part that Is affected. This is very effective.

Rub the affected part also with milk and olive oil. This is very effective.

Eat lot of protein diet for a good
growth and development of the skin.
This makes the worn out tissues to
be replaced by healthy skin tissues.

Protein food are fish, egg, beans,
peanuts and beef.

Eat Balanced Diet:

When a balanced diet is eaten, by
eating carbohydrate, protein,
unsaturated fatty acid (vegetable oil),

minerals, vitamins, iodized salt and water it makes the skin to be healthy and beautiful.

Eczema:

Eczema is treated by rubbing sliced lemon on the affected part.

Sliced lime can also be rubbed on the affected part.

Put thyme and curry into food when cooking. This is very effective.

Also take your bath in the morning

and in the night before going to bed

to sleep.

Petroleum Jelly(Vaseline).

It is good to be rubbed on the body

to prevent skin breakage.

It makes the skin to be radiant.

It makes the skin to be moisturized.

It makes the skin to be healthy and

beautiful.

Spinach:

This makes the skin to be beautiful.

It has antioxidant that protect the skin from free radicals that can damage the skin.

Use Of Body Lotion:

Use body lotion that is made from natural source that is healthy to the skin.

This moisturize the skin.

This makes the skin not to break.

This makes the skin to be soft.

This makes the skin to be beautiful.

Cracked Lips:

When there is cracked lips, drink enough water. This makes the skin to be hydrated.

Use olive oil to rub the lips.

Eat avocado and lettuce and cooked fish. This helps the cracked lips to become smooth and healthy.

The torn tissues, will be replaced by

healthy tissues.

This will make the place to be

beautiful and healthy.

Do Not Smoke.

Do not smoke. The smoke has free

radical that can cause damage to the

skin.

Do Not Use Recreational Drugs.

Recreational drugs can cause changes to the skin structure.

Recreational drugs can cause skin cancer.

Recreational drugs can cause skin cell necrosis(death).

Recreational drugs can be toxic to the skin.

Wear Neat Clothes.

Wearing neat clothes will prevent disease causing microorganisms from infecting the skin. This will

prevent disease of the skin, because

there will be no wearing of dirty

clothes that can cause pathogens

that may be in it to cause infection.

Vitamin A, vitamin C and vitamin E

are antioxidants that neutralize free

radicals that destroy skin cells. It is

therefore, good to eat fruits that are

having these vitamins. Such as

pawpaw, orange and vegetables.

Orange is used as an antioxidant, it

protect the skin from free radicals.

Orange is used on skin discoloration.

Ginseng

Ginseng is good for wound healing.

It is good for new growth of skin

cells.

Ginko is also good for healing of wound and the growth of new skin cells. It helps in the repair of worn out tissues.

Rosemary treat fungi infection and bacteria infection.

Rosemary treat pruritus(itching).

Rosemary treat acne.

Rosemary treat skin infections.

Sage:

Sage is used to treat acne.

It is also used to treat bacteria infection.

Parsley:

Parsley is used to moisturize the skin.

It is used as an astringent.

It is used to treat acne.

It is used to treat psoriasis.

It is used to treat eczema.

It is antiseptic.

Tea tree also treat fungi infection and bacteria infection.

Tea tree treat acne.

Tea tree treat viral infection.

Tea tree used to repel insects.

Bathing with soft sponge and mild soap makes the skin not to wear off.

Chamomile is used for itching skin. It

is also good to be used to treat

inflammation of the skin.

It is used as an antioxidant, it

protect the skin from free radicals.

It is used to heal traumatized skin

Citronella is used to repel insects.

Turmeric:

Put it into food that is going to be

cooked.

It helps as antibiotic to get rid of
disease causing microorganisms
from the skin.

It helps in the removal of dead
tissues from the skin.

When eaten with cooked fish it helps
in the replacement of dead tissues
with healthy tissues.

This makes the skin young and
beautiful.

It is used as antioxidant to prevent
damage of the skin by free radicals.

Remove Dirt From The Skin:

When ever the skin is dirty, it is good to wash that area with soap and water to make the area that is dirty to be clean. This prevent infection of that area by disease causing microorganisms.

Vitamin C:

Vitamin C prevent scurvy(itching of the eyes). This prevent scratching of the eyes. This prevent inflammation of the skin of the eye lead as a result of scratching. This makes redness, heat and swelling not to occur to the eye lead.

Vitamin E:

It is good to eat cooked green vegetables as soup. The vegetable oil in it makes fat not to accumulate inside the blood vessels(atherosclerosis), it makes fat plaque not to be in the heart. It makes the face not to be plumpy.

This makes the face to look young

and diseases are prevented.

Skin Rashes:

Skin rashes is prevented by bathing

in the morning and in the evening.

This prevent infection of the skin

that can cause rashes, because

pathogens that may be on the skin

that can cause rashes are washed

away from the skin. Therefore,

making the skin free from rashes.

Dandruff:

It is good to wash the head regularly

with soap and clean water. This

makes dandruff to be treated. It is

good to take bath regularly and

wash the head well with soap and

clean water for dandruff to be

prevented.

During A Sunny Day:

When you are outside during a sunny day, wear cap and use umbrella. This prevent skin cancer from ultra violet radiation. It also prevent redness of skin. It prevent skin burn. This makes the skin to be healthy and beautiful.

Use Mirror:

Use mirror to look at your face in order to examine it. This makes you to properly examine if there is any redness, swellings, acne, blackheads, pain and any infection and properly take good care of it so that the face can be healthy and beautiful. This also makes you to prevent infection.

Shoes:

Don't wear shoes that is too tight or too big. This prevent injury to the feet.

Keep your shoes clean this prevent infections from pathogens.

Wear socks before wearing your shoes, this prevent swelling of the feet and trauma(injury) to the feet.

Clean The House:

Clean the whole house. This prevent communicable diseases from affecting the skin.

Prevent Ionizing Radiation

Ionizing radiation, such as X-ray, gamma ray and ultraviolet ray can cause skin cancer formation.

Do not harm your skin, it can create way for bacteria, fungi and virus to infect the skin. It can cause spot to the skin. It can cause the skin to be disfigured.

Natural oil is good to be used on the skin. This makes the skin to be normal. It prevent changes in the color of the skin. It protect the skin

by inhibiting blisters.

Natural oil can be used daily and it

will not have negative reactions to

the skin.

It will protect the skin from breaking

and from been dehydrated.

It does not allow bacteria infection

of the skin.

It makes the skin to be well

nourished.

It prevent changes in the structure of the skin cells. It prevent inflammation of the skin. It is good for the natural oil not to have synthetic preservatives, synthetic additives, synthetic colorants, synthetic fragrance and things that are synthetic generally.

Synthetic substances can cause allergic reactions to the skin.

Synthetic preservatives can cause adverse effect to the skin.

Synthetic dyes can cause negative changes to the skin.

Synthetic additives can cause negative reactions to the skin.

Do not use dirty water to bath. It can cause infection to the skin due to the presence of pathogens. It can contain bacteria, viruses, fungi and other disease causing microorganisms.

In the case of poultry. After touching the fowls and feeding them it is expected for such person to take his or her bath. This will prevent any infection.

After exercise, it is expected for such person to take bath. This is because bacteria can act on the sweat and cause body odour. Taking of bath after exercise makes the skin to be clean.

It is good not to be close to places that are having high temperature.

For example, when baking bread in the oven. It is expected to leave the dough in the oven, and the person will be far from the oven until the dough is baked and the person can off the oven. Then the person can remove the baked bread from the oven. Staying long close to a high temperature area cause the skin to have hyperpigmentation. For a dark skin person, melanocytes will be produced excessively. This will make the skin to look darker in complexion.

Light skin will become redden in complexion.

High heat area can cause skin inflammation.

High heat area can cause skin burn.

It is good to take bath after leaving a high heat area. For example, after cooking or after baking.

It is good not to wear very thick close when the temperature as increased in the afternoon. And it is not good to wear very light clothes during a very cold whether. This makes the skin to be healthy and beautiful.

Conclusion

The skin is very healthy and beautiful when you drink clean water.

Eat well washed vegetables and fruits.

Do not drink synthetic drinks. Drink natural juice from fruits.

Do not drink alcohol.

Take your bath regularly in the morning and in the evening.

Do not eat animal fat.

Use vegetable oil in cooking.

Do not stay under the sun as an hobby.

Do exercise regularly.

Sleep well.

Make sure your clothes are clean.

Eat carbohydrates, protein, vegetables, fruits, whole cereals, fish, chicken, goat meat, ram meat, turkey, beef, egg, beans, liver and nuts moderately.

Use little salt in the food.

Do not use too much sugar in the food.

Do not have self medication. Go and see medical doctor in order for you to be healthy.

It is very good for parents to educate their children on how to take good care of the skin. This will prevent any adverse effect on the skin of the children.

It is very good to have clean environment. This prevent communicable diseases from affecting the parents and children.

www.ingramcontent.com/pod-product-compliance
Lightning Source LLC
Chambersburg PA
CBHW031137250726
48655CB00002B/722